MW01490542

Where Custom Smiles Are Created

Advanced Dental Care in One Location

Dr. Gary Silverstrom

Dr. David Silverstrom

SmartBox
819 Mount Tabor Road, Suite 300
New Albany, IN 47150
Toll Free: 888.741.1413
Fax: 502.371.0659
Email: colin@smartboxwebmarketing.com
Website: www.smartboxwebmarketing.com
Facebook: www.fb.me/SmartBoxWebMarketing
Twitter: @creceveur
YouTube: www.youtube.com/SmartBoxWeb

This book is not intended to replace the advice of a trained health professional. If you know or suspect you have a health problem, you should consult a health professional. The author and publisher disclaim any liability, loss, or risk, personal or otherwise, that is incurred directly or indirectly as a consequence of the use and application of the contents of this book.

Printed in the United States of America
First Printing, 2017

Contents

Why We Wrote This Book

DENTISTRY IS ABOUT MORE than filling cavities or polishing teeth. For us, dentistry is both life-changing and, in some cases, life-saving. Over the next several pages, you'll learn a little about our practice — The Silverstrom Group — what makes us different, and why we believe we're your next and final dental home.

The Silverstrom Group has been a Livingston, New Jersey, enterprise for more than 40 years. We are conveniently located just 20 miles west of Manhattan and treat patients from across the region. In that time, we have learned what's important to our dental patients. They want a great smile and treatments at a place that is convenient and state-of-the-art. To meet those expectations, we have built a modern facility that can treat patients of all ages and dental complications.

We're not a big corporate practice with hundreds of employees or patients that we consider "just another number." We have trained with leading experts around the world and have decades of experience under our belts. We also have a tight-knit staff with inspired local residents who genuinely love dentistry and their community. And, of course, every patient is treated like a member of our family. In fact, we would not suggest a treatment that we would not do for our own family members.

Our office uses some of the most advanced dental technology on the planet and even has an on-site lab where we build all our custom smile creations. In fact, our office mottos are "Where custom smiles are created" and "One tooth at a time." No other dentist in New Jersey has an on-site dental laboratory to achieve this level of personalization; rather, they rely on an outside lab to create restorations for "their" patients. We oversee every part of your dental procedures — nothing is outsourced. In many cases, you'll find that we can even treat major dental problems in one single visit. We're so confident in our work that everything comes with a 10-year guarantee.

Our Awards and Community Involvement

At The Silverstrom Group, we like to think that great dentistry can change the person and the community for the better. We're serious about our community involvement, so much that Dr. David Silverstrom received the prestigious Community Service Award from the Mayor of Livingston.

When it comes to our dental care, the results often

speak for themselves, but our patients have spoken on behalf of our treatments. We have been voted by patients as the best dentist by *Suburban Essex Magazine*'s readers for six years in a row. We were also given *New Jersey Monthly*'s Great Oak Award, which celebrates businesses focused on community services. The recipients of the Great Oak Awards are measured by their financial support and volunteerism.

One of our biggest ways of giving back is our devotion to cancer patients. Nearly everyone in this country knows someone affected by this terrible disease, and it's our job as medical professionals to help in any way we can.

Dr. David Silverstrom cofounded the New Jersey Makeover Team, made up of aesthetic medical professionals across the state. He is an ambassador, former board of director, and long-time supporter of the Mental Health Association of Essex County. In 2014, we both founded the Smiles for Life Award, which awards a full-mouth renovation to a cancer survivor. Cancer treatments like chemotherapy can wreak havoc on the mouth and cause patients to lose teeth or suffer with bad teeth. Each year, we partner with the American Cancer Society to provide a $25,000 cosmetic makeover to a cancer survivor. Here is a little more information about us.

Why I Became a Dentist
Dr. Gary Silverstrom

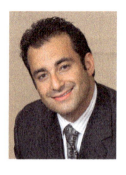

I believe there is no substitute for old-fashioned customer service and kindness. I love coming into the office every day and working with my hands to give someone a better smile. My father and I have worked hard to ensure that excellence is synonymous with the Silverstrom name.

It's safe to say that dentistry is part of my family. Being the son of a successful dentist inspired me to become a dentist, but I mostly discovered my love for dentistry in college. My friends all went into finance. That never appealed to me, and I kept coming back to dentistry. I quickly came to love the treatments, working with my hands, and, of course, the patient. My approach to dentistry is simple: I want to provide comfortable treatments and innovative technology for every patient and quickly resolve their dental issues. I care about the smile and the person behind the smile. I want to know your concerns, your smile goals, and any apprehensions you may have. I've never seen a smile that cannot be fixed, and I have countless hours of training in all disciplines of general dentistry. I'm certified in Invisalign, a leading clear orthodontic solution, and can provide computerized dentistry to give patients same-day crowns.

Some of my closest friendships started in our dental office.

I have attended countless weddings, bar mitzvahs, bat mitzvahs, birthdays, and graduations of my patients. I even had the distinct honor of being the wedding officiant for a patient. I'm sure that very few, if any, other dentists can say this! This person started out as a patient, but we developed a bond. Soon, we became close friends, and I was asked to officiate their wedding. I immediately accepted.

Why I Became a Dentist
Dr. David Silverstrom

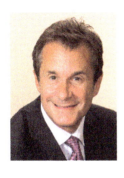

I wanted to become a dentist at an early age. To me, it seemed like the perfect way to help my community. When I started this career decades ago, I can still remember my excitement. To be honest, many years later, I still approach dentistry with the same vigor.

From the inception of The Silverstrom Group, I have worked to implement modern technology. It was important for me to find solutions that made our patients' visits more comfortable and pleasant. It's amazing the ways in which dentistry has advanced over the years. I love going to dental conferences around the country to train in new techniques and pick the brains of the industry's leading clinicians. This training has allowed me to introduce state-of-the-art treatments like laser cavity finders that

will detect even a speck of dental decay, dental implant placement, and advanced same-day crown services.
A career in dentistry has given me more than I ever could have imagined, and I get to practice with my son.

When it comes to treating patients, we focus on the benefits. We don't sell our patients any treatments, and we make sure they fully understand the benefits before moving forward with a procedure. We offer quick, pain-free treatments that can last you a lifetime!

Just by picking up this book, you might have found the solution to your dental problems. Here are a few things you'll learn:

- The importance of oral health and its relationship to your overall health

- How all-in-one dentistry means convenient, timely, and beautiful results

- How advanced technology can give you a better, brighter smile

- Why replacing missing teeth or fixing bad teeth can turn your life around

- What you can do to achieve a better smile or get back the smile you lost in your youth

CHAPTER 1

Your Next... and Final Dental Home

YOU WANT NATURAL TEETH THAT WILL LAST FOREVER.
You want that beautiful, bright smile.
You want to be without dental pain.
You don't want to be uncomfortable or afraid of the dentist.
You don't want those pesky gaps in your smile.
You want strong replacement teeth that will last forever.

You'll rarely find a dentist skilled in all aspects of dentistry. So, when something goes wrong, you'll likely find yourself driving all around town visiting dental experts whose names you'll never remember. You'll probably spend a great deal of your valuable time and hard-earned money.

The Silverstrom Group was established more than 40 years ago to fulfill each of these needs. We have helped hundreds of patients meet their smile goals with our comprehensive, custom, and gentle dental care.

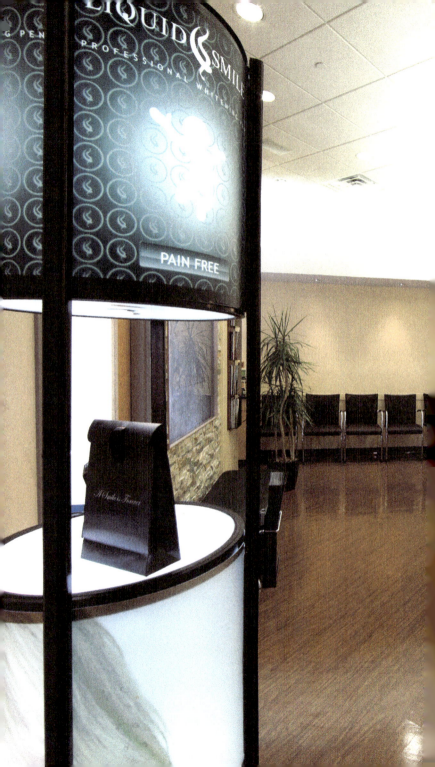

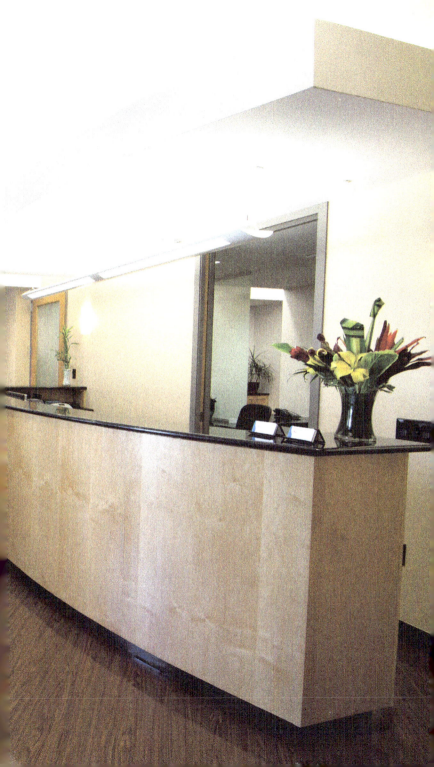

Both of us (Dr. David Silverstrom and Dr. Gary Silverstrom) have studied at the most elite dental institutions in the country and regularly attend continuing education around the world. Our dental careers, however, began not too far away at the New York University School of Dentistry. The school laid the groundwork for our dental skills and love of helping patients overcome their dental issues. But you certainly don't learn everything in dental school. Methods change and technology advances.

Some dentists are stuck in the dark ages of dentistry, and their patients suffer. Old techniques are often painful, time-consuming, and less effective, and outdated technology can lead to poor results. We stay on the cutting edge to treat patients' dental issues, big or small. We have advanced solutions to replace missing teeth, get you out of pain quickly, resolve those nagging cosmetic dental problems, and much more.

And then you have convenience...

At The Silverstrom Group, we bring the dentistry to you instead of asking you to go to specialists all around town. Everything is under one roof. And we mean *everything*, from the treatments to the state-of-the-art dental lab. We have the only on-site dental lab in New Jersey, and our master ceramists can design a custom smile at a moment's notice.

Dr. David Silverstrom launched our practice in 1977. Establishing a private practice was the dream of anyone who graduated from dental school in the 1970s. At that time, most dental practices were extremely similar, offering only general dentistry and using specialists for anything more.

The Silverstrom Group, however, was never your average dental office. Since we opened our doors, patients have received expert dental care in a modern, ever-evolving facility. Whenever a beneficial new procedure comes along, we learn it. Whenever we see an opportunity to implement effective new technology, we take it. Some of our staff members have worked with us for decades and have treated two or three generations of family members.

Around 2010, we asked ourselves how we could make the patient experience even better. So we created the Elle Jordan Studio, which lets us make beautiful, handcrafted restorations in-house. This way, we can oversee the entire process and make sure you're getting the best care you need.

Here are a few other things you'll find at The Silverstrom Group that you cannot expect at your average dental office:

Modern technology: 3D imaging (something you rarely find outside of a hospital) lets us precisely assess your mouth and plan treatments, especially when it comes to replacing teeth. This is made possible because of our cone beam computed tomography (CBCT).

Same-day smile solutions: Whether it's whitening

your teeth, repairing damaged teeth with crowns, or replacing all your teeth, we can often complete your entire dental treatment in a single visit.

Orthodontic solutions: Severe alignment or mildly crooked teeth aren't issues for us. We have options for everyone. One revolutionary orthodontic solution is Invisalign, a clear orthodontic system that gradually moves your teeth into a more appropriate position.

Laser dentistry: This is a great alternative to traditional oral surgery (especially for those with gum issues). Laser dentistry reduces tenderness and improves overall recovery.

Sedation dentistry: Still afraid of the dentist? No problem. Sedation dentistry can take the edge off and help you get the care you need.

Dental implants: Missing teeth or bad dentures? We can use dental implants, which nearly equal the strength of your natural teeth, to stabilize dentures or give you new permanent teeth. (You'll find out why these benefits are such a big deal later in the book.)

In-house specialists: You'll find specialists in every area of dentistry in our office. We have an in-office oral surgeon, a periodontist (gum specialist), an endodontist (addresses root problems), and multiple general dentists who are trained in all aspects of dentistry.

Care for the Entire Family

Part of being a one-stop shop means offering advanced treatments and *advanced* preventive treatments. We treat patients of all ages, whether they need cleanings or fillings. Just like with our advanced dental care, we have introduced digital technology to help with our preventive care. We have the laser cavity detectors that can locate even the slightest signs of decay and high-resolution intraoral cameras that we use to show you what's going on in your mouth.

And if your tooth needs a filling or other restoration, we have metal-free options that will blend in with your smile and function great for years to come.

One of the convenient things about our family dental practice is that we have multiple hygienists and doctors. This means parents can schedule the entire family for checkups on the same day. No more knocking off work multiple days just to get everyone in the family to their dental checkups.

Honoring Your Smile Goals

Perhaps the best way to learn about our office is to hear about people who have experienced our care. Being an all-in-one dental office, we have no "ideal" patients. We treat everyone, but following is one scenario we feel truly defines our office. This patient had substantial dental problems and needed help right away. She also shows what happens when you believe "one dentist is as good as the next."

A few months ago, a patient came into our office after struggling with bad teeth for years. She was embarrassed to smile. Some of her favorite foods were completely out of the question. The day-to-day misery was becoming too much for her to bear. She was wearing partial dentures to fill the gaps in her smile, and she constantly had to use denture adhesives. She needed a significant change. Like so many people, this patient — we'll call her Robin — didn't have great dental care as a child, and her teeth paid the price later in life. Robin also didn't have a good grasp of modern dentistry. She thought one dentist was as good as the next. So she went to the dentist down the street to address her missing teeth. She did little research beforehand, so she didn't know about the new ways offices like ours can replace bad or missing teeth.

What happened is that she spent more time and money than she ever expected because she couldn't find the right dentist for her. At our office, we never disparage other practitioners, but every dentist certainly has their strengths and weaknesses.

In Robin's case, she visited a dentist who was not skilled in replacing missing teeth. That dentist's suggestions were a little outdated. So, she came to our office for help.

It turns out that she was dealing with a mouth of bad teeth. In one day, we removed eight teeth and placed four dental implants around her jaw. Our master ceramist crafted her new teeth to attach to the implants the same day as well. Robin walked out of our office feeling great about her smile and able to eat whatever she wanted again.

Robin is now happier than ever having fixed her mouth in a way that reflected her goals. As she discovered, the difference between our office and other offices is that we start with the patient's goals and then plan the treatment. It's nearly impossible to work the other way around.

This is just all in a day's work at The Silverstrom Group. Robin's story is typical, not the exception.

Great Dentistry Means a Healthier Life

Why are we so focused on cutting-edge dentistry? Easy. It means better results and healthier mouths for our patients.

A patient's smile goals are of the utmost importance to the dental team at The Silverstrom Group. We never complete a procedure unless the patient understands the specifics. Honoring personal smile goals is one thing, but improving your appearance is not our only benefit to you. A great dental professional can give you a beautiful smile while also improving your oral and overall health.

You see, a healthy smile is imperative. Dental diseases or bad teeth can take a toll on your body. For example, gum disease, also known as periodontal disease, is one of the most prevalent diseases on the planet and the leading cause of tooth loss. If left untreated, gum disease can spread throughout your mouth and, to make it worse, has been connected to issues like diabetes and heart disease. While there is no known cause and effect, we do know that people with gum disease are more likely to have diabetes and heart disease. Plus, gum disease brings on issues like inflammation and bleeding, things you definitely don't want to experience on a daily basis.

You'll read a great deal about gum disease throughout the book, as it's something we dentists spend a lot of time worrying about, treating, and helping our patients avoid. In our office, we have the ability to treat your gum disease with noninvasive procedures, but we'll have much more on that later.

There are many more ways in which a healthier mouth can give you better overall health.

Healthy gums means a healthier diet. Gum disease is the number one cause of tooth loss. When you experience tooth loss, it's hard to eat the nutritious foods you need, and studies show that people without teeth can die earlier than those with teeth.

Removing any abnormalities can reduce your risk

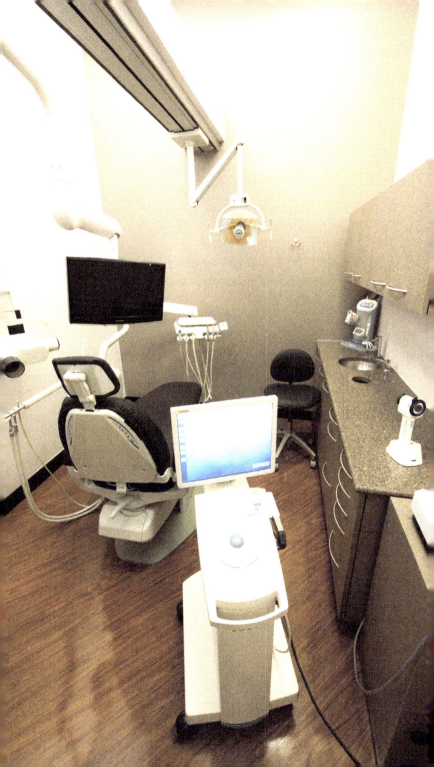

of cancer. During your examinations, we're doing much more than looking for cavities and gum disease. A dentist serves as the first (and often only) line of defense in detecting problems like oral cancer. Oral cancer is treatable if caught early, but the survival rate is grim if the problem is caught in its later stages. And it doesn't just affect those who smoke or use tobacco. A percentage of oral cancer cases are not tied to any known cause.

Treating TMD (temporomandibular joint disorder) means relieving headaches and neck pains. Patients who grind or clench their teeth, particularly due to an uneven bite, often have TMD. It leaves them at risk of wearing down or fracturing teeth. People with untreated TMD frequently wake up with headaches, stiff necks, and even back pain because they grind or clench their teeth during sleep.

Treating sleep apnea reduces risk of stroke and heart disease. Sleep apnea is a dangerous condition that occurs when people experience pauses in breathing while they sleep. There are reports of people having died in their sleep due to complications from sleep apnea. Untreated sleep apnea also increases your risk of problems like heart disease, stroke, diabetes, obesity, high blood pressure.

Straight teeth are easier to clean. Even something

as seemingly small as straightening your teeth makes it easier to clean your teeth and reduces the risk of tooth decay and gum disease.

These are just a few ways great dentistry can improve your overall health. Then you have problems occurring in your life that can wreak havoc on your smile:

A poor diet filled with carbohydrates and sugars (the worst cavity-causing foods)

Cola consumption (combination of acid and sugar)

Alcohol consumption (many alcohols are full of sugar)

Biting nails/chewing on ice (adds stress to your teeth and increases their risk of fracturing)

Persistent dry mouth (allows plaque and bacteria to attack teeth and gums)

Tooth grinding/clenching (puts wear and tear on your teeth and gums)

Smoking (tobacco stains the teeth and increases risk of gum disease and tooth decay)

Skipping dental appointments (small problems can develop into major problems when you don't maintain regular appointments; chapter 5 is devoted to addressing what causes people to skip their appointments)

As you can see, your daily habits can affect your oral health, *and* your oral health can affect your overall health. It's a deep connection that should not be taken lightly. That's why whenever we suggest treatments, we do something called a Risk Assessment Profile. This profile is 100 percent unique to you. The profile assesses what will happen if you get treatment versus forgo treatment.

It's hard to live a great, happy life without a great dental professional in your corner. We love to coach patients on their health, console them about their problems, and, best of all, provide lifelong solutions.

Just hear from our patients who have partnered with us to save their teeth, replace their teeth, or get out of pain. Our website has hundreds of five-star reviews from happy patients. Following is just one of those reviews. Notice how this patient took the "typical route" of visiting numerous general dentists and specialists to resolve his many issues. What happened is that no one was truly coordinating his treatment. Here is more from him.

> *After spending tens of thousands of dollars on two orthodontists, three periodontists, three oral surgeons, and five general dentists, I went to Dr. Silverstrom. He was not only able to rescue my teeth from periodontal disease, but he provided me with the ability to smile openly after*

years of hiding my teeth. What sets Dr. Silverstrom apart from the other professionals I have encountered is his concern for his patients in addition to his superior technical knowledge of dentistry. He has a practical, caring approach to treating his patients. His staff reflects this practical, caring approach as well. Their main concern is for the patient's well-being. They are extremely professional in all aspects of patient care as well as the practical and economic perspective of each patient. Additionally, they reflect the same concern for patient comfort. I highly recommend this practice. You will receive not only the best dentistry but you will get a caring, pragmatic approach to your treatment as well.

CHAPTER 2

Take Your Dental Care to the Next Level

IT'S ONE THING to attract new patients; it's entirely different to keep patients for 10 years, 20 years, 30 years, or even 40 years! There are some patients who have been with The Silverstrom Group since we opened. A huge reason for this is the dedicated staff, but our patients also have come to expect advanced treatments, technology, and convenience.

There is an old adage: "If the only tool you have is a hammer, everything looks like a nail." Of course, hammers and nails have no place in dentistry, but some dentists are still generations behind on their tools and treatments. They are using the same methods they learned in dental school, even if they do the required dental continuing education. Newer treatments and technology are much less invasive and lead to more accurate, predictable results. That's why we try to seek out and use the latest technology in every aspect of

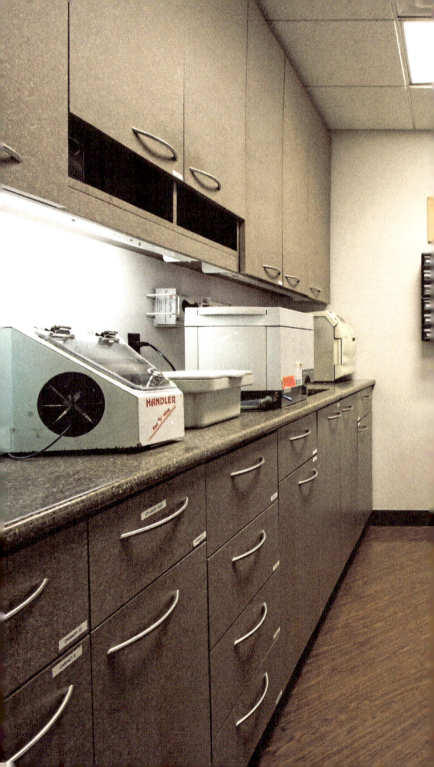

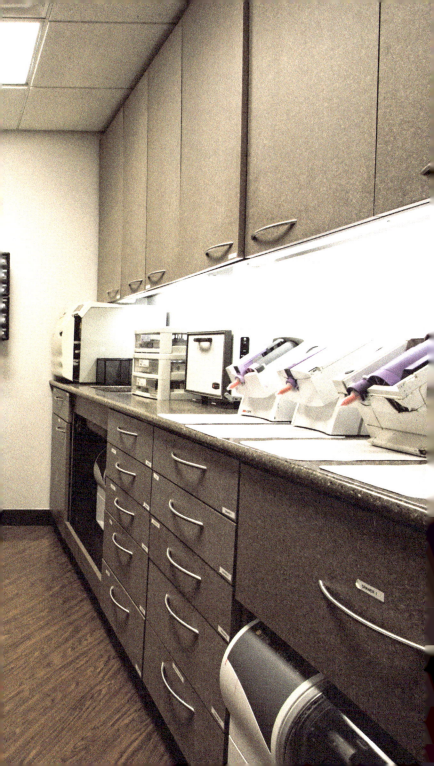

dentistry. This means everything from using advanced cameras to show the patient exactly what we see in their mouths to using advanced laser cavity detection equipment.

As you might imagine, we have many patients who have seen us transition to new technology over the years. Take Glenn, who has been a patient of ours for more than 35 years. He has had cosmetic and restorative treatments at our office, receiving everything from minor fillings to root canals and dental crowns.

Glenn was in one of the first groups of patients to benefit from our laser dentistry, same-day crowns, and even digital restoration imaging. He's been the beneficiary of almost every piece of modern technology at The Silverstrom Group. Here is how Glenn describes his experience at our practice and our cutting-edge technology.

What I feel that this group really represents is a desire to help the patient understand. I understand what they are going to do. I understand the options. I understand the implications. They make me part of the choice, part of the decision-making process, but they educate me in a way that I think is truly important to reach the right decision ... I've seen this practice grow and develop using new tools and new technology in ways that are really productive and helpful, not just for the dentist but for the patient's comfort.

Precise Dental Imaging
Means Better Results

Glenn's dental journey is different from most people's, but not most people who visit our office. He's had the benefit of not having to piecemeal his dental services. He's lucky. He's had the convenience most dental patients don't experience.

Having advanced technology isn't about having shiny objects around the office. As we touched on before, the technology improves your dental visits and overall treatment outcomes. In other words, it means comfort in the office and outside of the office.

Take 3D imaging. Few dental offices have the ability to take 3D images of your oral cavity. The Silverstrom Group has a cone beam computed tomography (CBCT) scanner that allows us to diagnose and plan dental treatments. The CBCT works by rotating around the head while taking hundreds of images of the teeth and oral cavity. The technology then converts these hundreds of images into 3D images. Obviously, 3D images allow us to take a closer look at what's going on in the mouth. Here are a few more advantages of CBCT technology:

• No uncomfortable film or X-ray material in your mouth

• Better diagnosis of dental problems

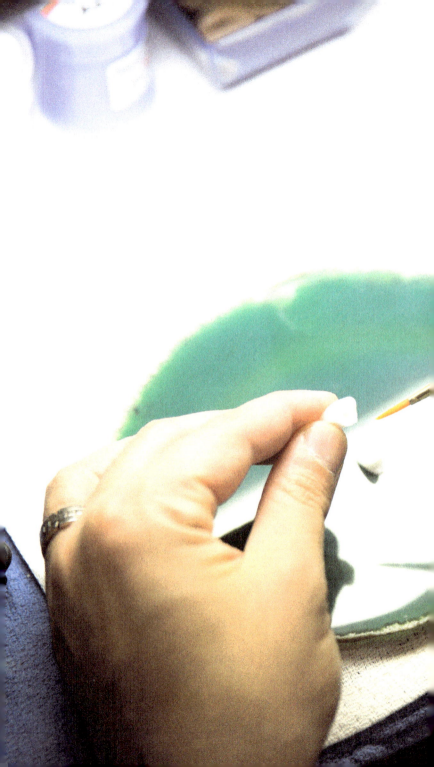

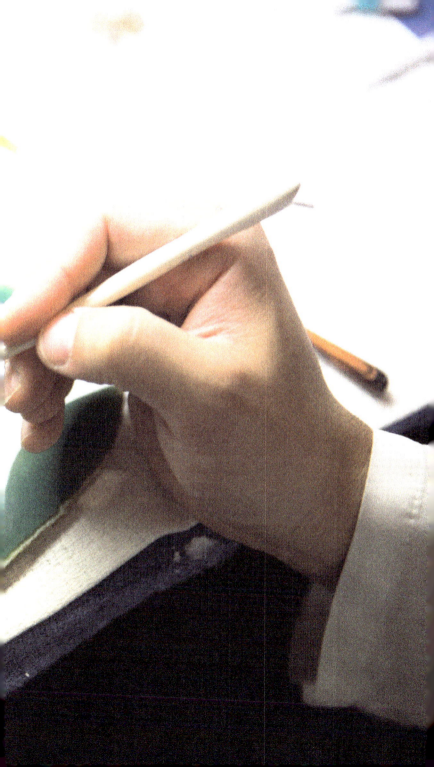

- Digital planning for advanced treatments like dental implant placement

- Reduction in overall oral surgery and recovery times

- Better results with preventive and restorative treatments

The CBCT is used in various ways, but perhaps one of its most beneficial uses is for placing dental implants. Dental implants have become the ultimate way to replace missing teeth. They are the strongest tooth replacement option available. As such, dental implants have become incredibly popular. Every dentist under the sun promotes dental implants, whether they offer the treatment or not. Some dentists say they offer dental implants, but they really only coordinate the treatment. So, if you need that implant, you'll be sent to a specialist for the actual procedure.

At The Silverstrom Group, we have placed dental implants for decades. To boot, each of our staff members completes more than 100 hours of continuing education a year. Using our CBCT technology, we can view the jawbone density and even the tiny blood vessels so we can find the most appropriate placement for dental implants. Your body has to accept the implants, and because the CBCT helps us in positioning the implant exactly where it should be, it increases the overall success of the treatment.

Important note: *You might think that dental implant placement is risky oral surgery, but that's far from the case. Dental implants can be placed with a more than 98 percent success rate.*

Restore Teeth in a Single Visit

A few years ago, Glenn walked into our office for a regular checkup. He had a tooth with a large filling that was growing weaker by the day. The filling was too big to drill out, so we recommended that Glenn restore the tooth with a dental crown. Like so many patients before that day (and many since), Glenn had expected the entire crown process to take three to four weeks — or even longer. He expected a temporary crown, multiple visits, and all the other hassles associated with the procedure. That drawn-out method of treatment has been used for decades, but we had something better and more convenient: same-day dental crowns.

At The Silverstrom Group, we have digital imaging and a special in-house milling system to give our patients a crown in just one trip here. A crown placement is one of the most common restorative dental procedures. Yet this typical procedure takes dentists multiple weeks to complete. We wanted something better for our patients, which is why we offer same-day dental crowns. There are many advantages to this process, other than obviously providing crowns in a single visit. What you gain from same-day crowns:

No terrible temporary crowns: Temporary crowns are necessary when the dentist cannot restore the tooth immediately. After the impression, the temporary crown serves as a placeholder until your permanent crown is ready. Temporary crowns are typically made from acrylic material that is neither lifelike or very functional. Worse yet, temporary crowns have a tendency to dislodge. That can be horrifying for patients and cause them to make yet another visit to the office.

No goopy impression material in your mouth: One of the worst parts about getting a crown is the impression. The goopy impression can be uncomfortable and trigger people's gag reflex. With computerized same-day crowns, there is no goopy material because everything is digital.

More accuracy: The life span of a crown has everything to do with the fit. Traditional impressions are often subject to human error. With our digital imaging, we perfectly scan the tooth to make sure we have the best fit for your crown.

Great-looking crowns: Much like the fit of the tooth, we can also perfectly match the shade of your natural smile.

The great thing about same-day dental crowns is that we can place multiple crowns in a single day. We can essentially rebuild your entire mouth in a few hours. Each crown will fit your smile perfectly and restore the health of your mouth.

Restore Your Mouth with Laser-Assisted, Pain-Free Treatment

You read earlier that gum disease is the leading cause of tooth loss in adults. It's also extremely prevalent — affecting about 75 percent of adults in America. With something so bad and so common, we need a great, pain-free treatment to combat the negative effects of gum disease. This is where laser dentistry comes into play.

Let's go back to Glenn's story for a moment. The Silverstrom Group was an early adapter of laser technology, and Glenn was one of our first patients to benefit from laser dentistry. Laser dentistry has become one of our best defenses against harmful gum disease. When gum disease is in its advanced stages, the gums begin to separate from the teeth, creating infectious pockets. The traditional way to treat this is through scaling and root planing. For this process, we remove the tartar and bacteria buildup from under the tooth and gums and clean out the infection in these pockets.

The laser uses focused light to evaporate the infection in the periodontal pocket. It also allows for the teeth and gums to naturally reattach. Here are a few other major benefits of laser gum treatment:

Pain-free dentistry: Traditional gum surgery requires the use of scalpels and stitches. Basically, the dentist or periodontist — a gum specialist — will actually cut the infection out of the mouth. Laser dentistry doesn't rely on this method and instead evaporates the infection.

Less recovery time: This is a common benefit of any of our technology. Because we don't need to use scalpels or stitches, you'll experience less sensitivity after the procedure. Additionally, because the gums and teeth naturally reattach with the laser, there is less chance of infection.

Faster procedure: With laser dentistry, you can be in and out of the office much faster than with traditional gum surgery. There are fewer steps in the process, and we don't have to stitch the gums after the treatment.

More accurate treatment: The laser treatment is precise and effectively targets the infection. Instead of cutting away at the gums, the treatment is focused.

Many people can't wait around to treat their problems. Gum disease typically begins small — with bleeding or swollen gums — but can develop into a full-blown dental crisis if left untreated. If you have signs of gum disease or a history of gum disease, you need treatment that is precise and comfortable. Laser dentistry is that answer for many patients who come to The Silverstrom Group.

Straighten Teeth Without Braces

Most cavities aren't visible when you smile. And other people can't feel your dental discomfort. But people can definitely see your alignment issues. A recent study by Kelton Global found that the smile is the most important thing when it comes to making a good first impression. So a smile means more than your hair or even the clothes you wear. That's one of the major reasons The Silverstrom Group studies every feasible way to improve the smile.

When it comes to misaligned teeth, we have a great tool for patients of all ages: Invisalign. We are certified to provide teens and adults with Invisalign and have helped countless patients using this orthodontic method. This treatment has no metal brackets and no wires. Instead, it uses plastic aligners that are virtually invisible. The series of aligners gradually move teeth into a better position.

An Invisalign treatment typically takes anywhere from 12 to 18 months — about half the time of traditional braces. Patients who choose Invisalign also enjoy the freedom of having a removable appliance instead of something cemented to their teeth. You'll simply remove the Invisalign trays for eating, cleaning, and special occasions.

Speaking of eating, you can eat whatever you want with Invisalign. People with braces have to avoid delicious foods like steak, corn on the cob, popcorn, and more. But with Invisalign, you just remove the aligners during your meals, give your teeth a good brushing afterward, and then place the aligners back into your mouth. Just be sure to wear these aligners for at least 20 to 22 hours a day.

Invisalign's benefits don't stop there, though. Invisalign trays are comfortable and will not irritate the soft tissue in your mouth like traditional braces can. Invisalign patients love seeing their teeth transform right before their eyes, and they also love how discreet the treatment is. People can't see the trays, and they will not affect your speech. No one but you will need to know that you're fixing your teeth!

Comfortable, Safe Dentistry with Sedation

A few decades ago, the fearful dental patient didn't have many options. They either had to grit their teeth and bear their dental fear or succumb to their fear — which typically meant avoiding the dentist at all costs. At The Silverstrom Group, we pride ourselves on our friendly and professional staff. From the time you call to the moment we start your treatment, we aim to make you as comfortable as possible. That's why we have a relaxing dental spa atmosphere that includes incredible amenities for each patient who walks through the doors. Part of your dental spa experience includes complimentary refreshments and coffee, on-demand video, reading material, hot towels, aromatherapy, and a special relaxation room.

You can expect our treatments to be gentle and non-invasive, but we also have a special weapon to help patients battle dental fear: dental sedation!

Dental sedation comes in many different levels, and we offer them all, from nitrous oxide to general anesthesia. The first level of sedation, nitrous oxide, works quickly and wears off quickly. This is great for the mildly anxious patient. Then, you have the deepest levels of sedation, IV sedation and general anesthesia. Our office has a board certified anesthesiologist who can render sedation for fearful patients or those patients who need a full-mouth reconstruction.

Because we are a full-service dental office focused on restoring mouths, we often use sedation for patients who need longer appointments. Let's assume you need several dental implants (we'll get into the different implant treatments later). That can be a long process that requires a lot of appointments. With sedation dentistry, we can set up your treatment for one single day. That means fewer visits and fewer times you'll need to be numbed for the procedures.

Sedation dentistry is perfectly safe, and with a heavy level of sedation, you won't have to experience the sights, sounds, or smells of the procedures. These three S's are often the biggest contributors to dental fear.

At The Silverstrom Group, technology helps us give you precise results while educating you about your treatment. Remember Glenn? All of his dental treatments helped him get a better smile, but the technology also helped him make informed decisions about his health.

CHAPTER 3

Missing Teeth: How You Got Here and What to Do Next

THERE ARE MILLIONS OF AMERICANS who struggle with missing teeth. The problem takes a toll on your body, mind, and spirit, and worse, you're reminded of this misfortune several times a day … every time you eat, speak, smile, or laugh.

Your teeth are meant to last forever. They serve an important purpose in digesting food and maintaining a healthy diet. In this chapter, we want to show you the far-reaching problems of missing teeth — and introduce the solutions we offer to resolve these problems for good.

Having failing teeth can cause extreme pain and discomfort in your mouth, and losing your teeth can also be uncomfortable — and traumatic as well. And then you have the aftereffects of losing your teeth. Simply put, when teeth are lost, you have much more to worry about than how you look. It's a lifelong struggle.

If you are already dealing with bad or missing teeth, you get it. You don't need a lecture from us. But know that we have patients who have been right where you are. For example, we have an excellent patient named Janet. She came to The Silverstrom Group a few years ago after having worn removable dentures for several years. Janet's dentures made everything a challenge. She worried about her teeth every time she bit into something, and she had to reapply an uncomfortable denture adhesive multiple times a day. When she came to our office, she joked that she used so much denture adhesive over the years that she should have invested in the company. There are literally millions of people in this country just like Janet. We actually treat "Janets" all the time. We have heard just about every denture complaint in the book:

> *My dentures don't allow me to eat the food I want.*
> *My dentures wobble around in my mouth.*
> *My dentures don't look right.*
> *My dentures are warped and no longer have a snug fit.*
> *My dentures are uncomfortable and create sores in my mouth.*
> *I hate the messy denture adhesive.*
> *I'm worried that if I laugh or eat in public that my dentures will fall out.*

The last complaint is the most common. People who lose their teeth believe that removable dentures can restore their mouth. That, unfortunately, isn't the case. Removable dentures restore your biting force to only a fraction of what it was with natural teeth. People with traditional removable dentures have only between 25 and 50 percent of the power of natural teeth.

Take a look at these pictures of dentures. You can see why conventional dentures are hard to keep in your mouth. The lower denture rests on the gums, allowing it to shift around. Meanwhile, the upper denture covers the roof of the mouth, blocking some tastes and sensations.

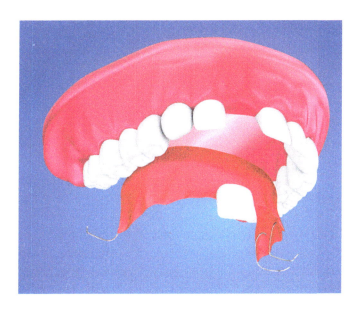

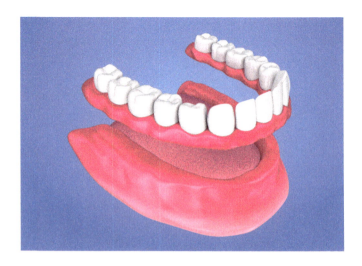

Not being able to eat the food you love is one thing, but having missing teeth or failing teeth can also create some serious health problems.

According to the world-renowned Mayo Clinic, people who have their natural teeth can live an average of **10 years** longer than those who do not have their teeth. It's safe to say that having missing teeth is an overall health crisis.

Where It All Begins

To understand the issue of missing teeth, you need to find the source of the problem. As it happens, most teeth fail because of gum issues, specifically gum disease. You read about this earlier in the book, but it bears repeating: Gum disease is the number one cause of tooth loss. This problem will affect about 75 percent of Americans at some point. It's of epidemic proportions, and it can quickly take over your mouth.

Unlike other epidemics in this country, however, most people are ignorant of the harmful effects of gum disease. They go about their lives without a clue that this problem might be lurking under the surface. But sooner or later, it rears its ugly head and can do some serious damage to your mouth.

Gum disease, also known as periodontal disease, occurs when bacteria accumulates to cause inflammation of the gums. There are two basic stages of gum disease, gingivitis and periodontitis, with periodontitis being the severe form. Gingivitis can be reversed with dental intervention, but periodontitis is a lifelong problem that will need constant care.

What Claims Your Teeth

While about 75 percent of Americans will suffer from gum disease at some point, about 10 to 15 of that population will have periodontitis. That's still millions of people to worry about. People in this stage often lose one tooth, multiple teeth, or all of their teeth. It can happen fast, too.

First, the bacteria will make its way into the gums, harboring there until it causes inflammation and bleeding. Next, what's known as periodontal pockets form.

As we alluded to earlier, these infectious pockets develop between the teeth and the gums, causing the gums to pull away from the teeth. The process will continue throughout the mouth. Ultimately, the infection reaches the bone, causing it to deteriorate. People who lose teeth because of gum disease do so because the tooth, no longer supported by sufficient bone or gum tissue, becomes loose in the socket. Once the tooth is loose, it's hard to save.

And the problems don't stop there.

Why the Jawbone Recedes

Your teeth are anchored by your jawbone, so when you lose teeth, your jawbone will change shape. This happens whether you lose a single tooth, a few teeth, or all your teeth.

Jawbone deterioration can cause the remaining healthy teeth in your mouth to shift around. But one of the most stunning effects of jawbone recession is that your facial structure will change. Think about it: your jawbone helps shape your face. If that bone recedes, your face structure will change. If you're wearing a removable appliance, the constant changes in the jawbone make it next to impossible for your appliance to fit perfectly.

Most notably, you'll lose the vertical height between your nose and chin. This is distracting and makes you look older than you are. In fact, before they replaced their teeth, some of our patients told us that their missing teeth and jawbone recession made them look and feel 10 years older.

At The Silverstrom Group, we have worked with many patients struggling with tooth loss, and we can attest that having no teeth or gaps in your smile substantially changes your appearance. Not only that, but people often have to change their diets when they lose teeth. Most foods that are hard, sticky, or crunchy are suddenly off the menu. You simply cannot get the power behind your bite to eat a variety of foods when your teeth are gone. You also lose the ability to chew and digest a variety of foods, including healthy foods like fruits, vegetables, and nuts (or the foods people love to eat, like pizza and steak!).

What to Do About Missing Teeth

You've read a lot of information about how missing teeth affect your everyday life. Many people know these problems firsthand and don't need a reminder. It's not our intent to pick out flaws in your smile without providing solutions, but we've found that understanding the risks of missing teeth helps people make informed decisions about how to treat the problem.

There is no better way to replace missing teeth than dental implants. Dental implants not only are strong and long-lasting; they can also be placed anywhere in the mouth. Dental implants are the ideal treatment for patients with one missing tooth or a mouthful of missing teeth.

At The Silverstrom Group, we use dental implants to give patients their smiles back and restore their confidence. It's our mission to give every patient a beautiful, strong smile, and dental implants are one tool that helps us accomplish this. Read on to learn about the specific benefits of dental implants, why patients love them, and, best of all, how you can come to The Silverstrom Group with a mouthful of failing teeth — or no teeth at all — and leave with teeth that can last forever.

CHAPTER 4

Teeth That Will Outlive You: Dental Implants

A FEW TITANIUM RODS, a few hours, and a few dental professionals can change your life. That's the basic formula for placing dental implants to replace your missing or failing teeth. Dental implants are not a temporary solution to a major problem. They can last a lifetime and all but make you forget that you lost your natural teeth. You'll feel like a new person who has a carefree, more youthful smile and can eat whatever you so choose.

With something so advantageous, you might assume that any dentist would offer this solution. But that's not the case. More and more dentists *are* offering dental implants, but few dental offices have the full spectrum of dental implants that you'll find at The Silverstrom Group.

Placing dental implants requires a blend of science, technology, technique, and artistry. The procedure has

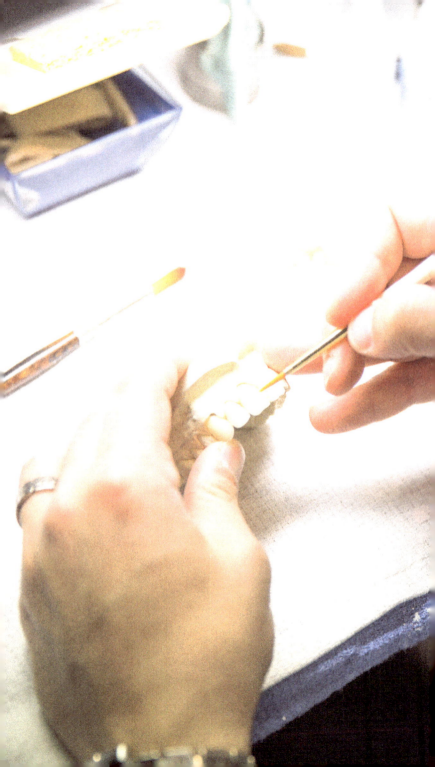

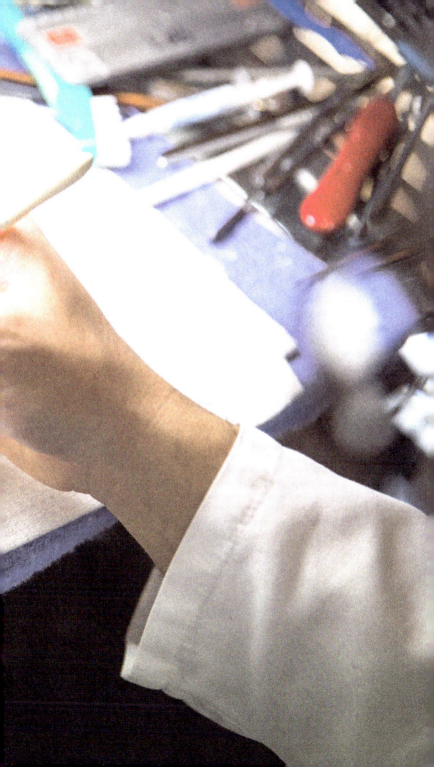

evolved for decades, so much that at The Silverstrom Group we can now place dental implants in a single visit. You can visit our office with a mouth full of terrible, failing teeth and leave with teeth that are strong and can last forever.

We've come a long way since dental implants were first introduced by dentists in the 1960s. The original implants, called "blade implants," worked only about 50 percent of the time. Today, we can place dental implants with a 98 percent success rate. So, don't get lost obsessing over dental implant placement being oral surgery. The treatment is highly successful, and once it's completed, you should never have to worry about your teeth again.

Dental implants can help nearly any patient with missing teeth. It doesn't even matter how you lost your teeth. Dental implants work for patients who lose their teeth because of gum disease, cavities, and root issues, as well as those who experience dental trauma or have congenital tooth loss. Some of our dental implant patients wore dentures for years, while others needed a quick and unexpected tooth replacement option.

One of our patients, Robert, struggled with bad dentures for years. He got upper and lower dentures after his teeth were claimed by poor oral hygiene and gum disease. Robert's dentures severely limited his food options and caused him to develop sores around his mouth. His dentures wobbled around, and like most denture wearers, he was terrified that they would fall

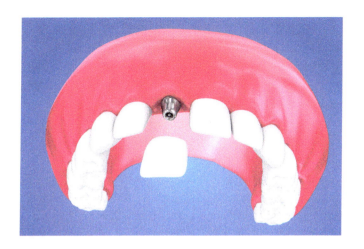

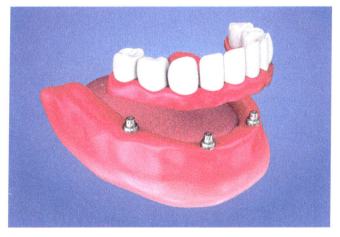

out of his mouth whenever he laughed or ate his food. You know from reading previous chapters that the longer you go without teeth, the harder it is to restore your mouth. In Robert's case, he had lost a significant portion of his jawbone structure, which further limited his food options.

When Robert came to The Silverstrom Group, he was living on a bland, soft-food diet and applying denture adhesives several times a day. Robert was ready to toss his dentures in the trash and go without teeth forever. When he visited our office, he was surprised to hear us encourage him to do just that! We hate dentures for the very reason our patients hate dentures: they can be impossible, especially the lower denture. The upper denture relies more on suction, while the lower denture relies more on fit. Physical changes like jawbone recession can affect both of these. Dentures are challenging for patients, and we hate seeing our patients struggle with something so vital to their health and happiness. Dental implants are a substantial investment, but the value overwhelmingly outweighs the cost.

We mentioned earlier that dental implants are one of the most versatile tools used in dentistry. After we encouraged our patient Robert to throw away his dentures, we steered him toward dental implants that are restored with bridge-like teeth that cannot be removed. This method is called All-on-4® dental implants. The process is simple: we place a series of four dental implants around the jaw and restore those implants with new, nonremovable teeth. One of the best parts about the All-on-4 process is that the upper palate is not covered, giving the patient more tastes and hot and cold sensations. This is music to a patient's ear, as traditional dentures cover the roof of the mouth and can obstruct taste buds.

Before receiving his All-on-4 dental implants, Robert couldn't eat some of his favorite foods: steak, nuts, and fresh fruits and vegetables. Within a few days of receiving his dental implants, Robert had eaten all of these foods. At that point, he had gone years without much of his favorite treats. He continues to enjoy his favorite foods without concern of his teeth dislodging or wobbling around.

The Silverstrom Group has offered dental implants for several decades, and we have always stayed on the cutting edge. We have also treated just about every type of patient you can imagine. Robert represents just some of the patients who come to us struggling with dentures. We've helped people with much more severe bone loss than Robert's, and of course, those who had only one or a few missing teeth. So, if you've been thinking your smile isn't fixable, let us stop you right there. Modern dentistry and tools like dental implants allow us to fix just about anything. We'll show you how your smile can change during a consultation at our office.

How Our Dental Implants Work

Dental implants are so successful because we use material that is compatible with your body. Each dental implant is made from a tiny, screw-like piece of titanium. Researchers in the 1950s unintentionally discovered that titanium fuses to bone, and it wasn't too long until titanium was used for the first dental implants. The newest dental implants are made from threaded titanium screws and are placed carefully in- the jawbone. The process of titanium merging with bone is called osseointegration, which is just a fancy way to say that the implant literally becomes part of your body.

Here's a basic breakdown of the implant process. First, we remove any failing teeth that need to come out. If we can address missing teeth right away, we can almost always forgo bone or gum grafting. If it's been awhile since the natural tooth has been removed, we might recommended some grafting to build up the jawbone to support the implant.

Next, we place the dental implant. Unless we are placing the tooth directly into an old tooth socket, we'll use special 3D imaging to find the most appropriate locations for the implants. Just to remind you, few dental offices have 3D imaging capability. Because this technology helps us find the best location for each implant, it reduces sensitivity and improves the implant's overall success rate. We typically place dental implants under mild sedation or simply local anesthesia. If you are prone to dental anxiety — or if you need extensive dental work — we might suggest general anesthesia. We have an anesthesiologist on staff to handle all your dental sedation needs.

The second to last step is waiting for the implant to heal. While we can place and restore dental implants in a single day, we usually wait for the implant to heal around the bone before we place the final restoration.

Last of all, we'll place your permanent restoration. We have a dental laboratory in-house where we create handcrafted restorations to perfectly fit your smile. Our dental lab, Elle Jordan Studio, is vital in giving you a great dental experience. We don't have to send your impressions to an outside lab to fabricate your restoration. This cuts down on the wait and gives you precise results.

Implants Are for Everyone

Every titanium dental implant functions in a similar way, but not every dental implant system is the same. It takes extensive training and updated technology to meet different implant needs. Some patients have different goals or needs than other patients. For example, if you are missing entire arches of teeth, we can retrofit your dentures to attach to implants or use the All-on-4 dental implant method.

The difference between All-on-4 dental implants and implant-secured dentures is that All-on-4 restorations are not dentures. All-on-4 teeth can only be removed by a dentist, while implant-secured dentures can be removed by the patient for easy cleaning.

Then there's Teeth in a Day®. This is when we can remove failing teeth and place dental implants in a single visit. The entire process only takes about 90 minutes, and you won't have to go without teeth. This treatment is particularly beneficial because many dentists who offer dental implants extract the failing teeth and then have the patient wait a few weeks until they place the dental implants. That's weeks you'll spend without teeth and without smiling — and perhaps worst of all, everyone you know and anyone you bump into will see your dental history on display.

At The Silverstrom Group, we make sure you are never without teeth. Additionally, each dental implant we place carries a 10-year guarantee. If anything goes wrong within that period, just visit us again and we'll fix your problem for free, as long as you maintain your oral health as we've advised.

When you visit The Silverstrom Group for your dental implant services, you'll be treated like a member of the family. You'll experience our comfortable office and pain-free dental solutions. You'll be eating and smiling again without restraint in no time. And you could even turn back the clock on your appearance, giving you a fuller and more youthful smile.

CHAPTER 5

The One Thing You Won't Have at The Silverstrom Group: Fear!

WE'VE MENTIONED several advanced procedures in this book. We've written in depth about how dental implants, tooth extractions, digital technology, same-day crowns, and Invisalign can help your smile. Some of these treatment concepts may be new for you, and therefore a little intimidating. Or maybe you have a sour view of dentistry and hate going to the dentist. We understand the impulse to fear certain treatments or some aspects of dentistry, but don't let your preconceived notions about dentistry get in the way of your health.

For one, the old methods of treating dental problems are a thing of the past — at least at The Silverstrom Group. Forget everything you think you know about the sights, sounds, and smells of dentistry. This is not your father's or grandfather's dental office. Our modern dental procedures save you time and, in many cases, are pain-free. Every tool — from our laser dentistry to our 3D imaging — is here to increase the overall success of your treatment and minimize or eliminate discomfort!

At The Silverstrom Group, our patients continue coming back because we have left no stone unturned when it comes to patient comfort. We have a TV in each operatory, complimentary refreshments from our Silverstrom Cafe, warm towels, and even a relaxing meditation room with aromatherapy options. And perhaps best of all, we are a lecture-free, guilt-free zone. We'll never make you feel bad about your smile, regardless of your dental condition.

Of course, not all dental offices are like this. And it would be naive to think that every dental fear is unfounded. But first, let's examine what dental fear is and its causes.

There are literally millions of Americans who skip their dental appointments out of fear. Dental organizations estimate that about 9 to 15 percent of Americans avoid the dentist at all costs (this means no cleanings, checkups … nothing). Most people have a mild anxiety about the dentist, especially when dealing with a new treatment. That's perfectly normal, and it can be helped with a caring voice or quick meet-and-greet with a friendly dentist.

Dental anxiety is extremely common, but dental phobia is a different beast entirely. Dental phobia can be unfounded or caused by a bad previous experience at the dentist. We have met people who have suffered immensely at the hands of a dentist earlier in their lives. Then there are the people who cringe even picturing the dental equipment or imagining the sounds in the office. Frankly, we also see a lot of patients who have lost faith in dentistry altogether. They have spent years visiting different dentists and having a host of procedures that never turned out the way they wanted. We're here for those patients as well, and we hope those patients don't give up on the chance to have beautiful, functional smiles.

It's our goal at The Silverstrom Group to make sure we never contribute to someone's dental phobia. Far from it. We aim to cure it!

The Silverstrom Group takes pride in helping patients overcome their dental fears while also giving them a smile that will withstand the test of time. We've treated generations of family members, and it's not unusual to see patients we've had for 10 years, 20 years, or even 30 years or longer.

Our dedicated patients are a testament to our ability to provide pain-free, stress-free care. Take our patient Ellen. She has been coming to our office for more than 25 years. When she first came here, we wouldn't exactly say she was enthusiastic about the dentist. Over her time with us, she has had just about every dental treatment you can think of. Today, she has a great smile that will last her the rest of her life. When we asked her to give us one reason she visits our office, she didn't

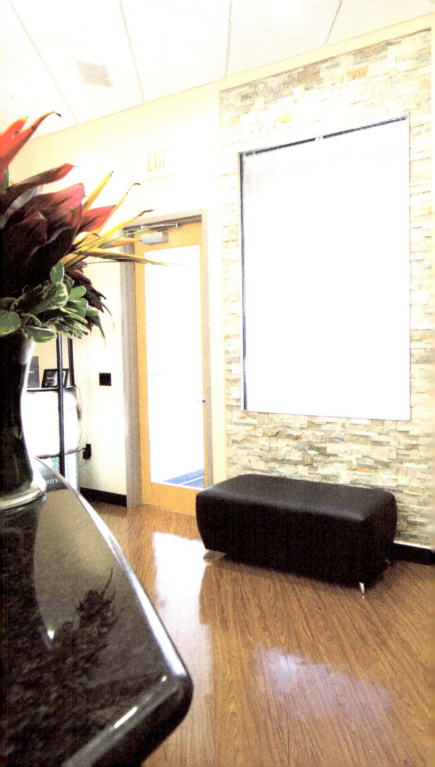

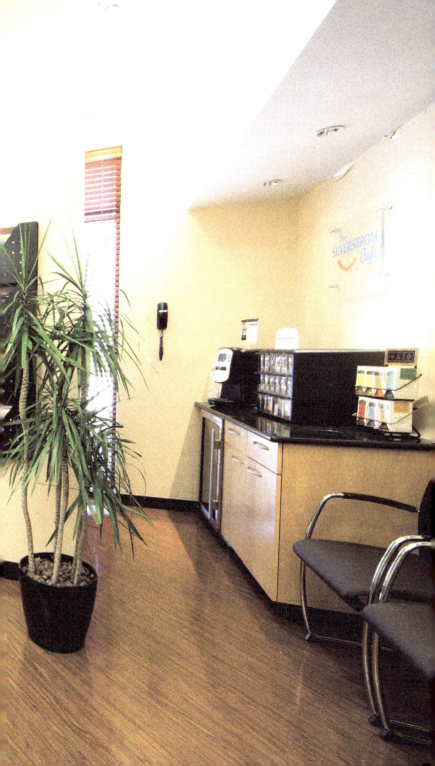

mention the procedures at all. Instead, she said it was about her connection with us and the dental team.

Probably the number one reason I have been coming to (Dr.) David (Silverstrom) and his group for the past 25 years can be summed up in one word: trust. I can trust him to take care of me, to do exactly what he tells me he's going to do. I know what to expect, and it happens. He never hurts me. He has always promised me that he would never hurt me and he never has! … I never feel that I'm being pressured into any procedure; it just isn't the way they do business here.

Education and Technology Goes a Long Way

During a casual stroll through our office, you'll quickly notice the number of high-tech machines and digital tools we use. As we've touched on, The Silverstrom Group doesn't look or function like your typical dental office. We have invested in the right digital tools to aid us in effectively diagnosing your dental problems and setting up the necessary treatments.

Easing dental fear often starts with teaching. Our digital tools like intraoral cameras and 3D imaging can show patients what we see inside their mouths. Using the intraoral camera, we'll actually show you what your teeth and gums look like in real time. This way, we can show you what decay looks like or just better explain what areas of your mouth need attention. Patients tend to relax once they understand what we're looking at or working on in their mouths.

The 3D imaging is perhaps our most important resource when it comes to diagnosing and planning treatments. The detailed images also allows you to better understand the procedure. If we are placing dental implants, we can use our 3D digital technology to show you every step of the procedure. We'll show you exactly where the implants will go and what your smile will look like once the procedure is finished.

When we take patients aside before starting treatment and show them the results using our advanced technology, they are much more likely to understand the treatment. Additionally, they won't have any surprises about what the procedure is, or the outcome. And as you now know, our in-house dental laboratory, Elle Jordan Studio, eliminates weeks or even months from your overall treatment time. You can meet your ceramist and have your smile rebuilt in just one day.

The Next Level of Relaxation

Being comfortable in the dental chair is half the battle. Patients need to be comfortable and confident before we start any procedure. Earlier, we made a distinction between dental anxiety and dental phobia. Unfortunately, some people cannot be helped or comforted just by seeing a friendly face or understanding how our technology can make their treatments stress-free. They need something more. This is why we offer sedation dentistry. Sedation is one of the easiest ways to help patients relax in the chair. It's safe, and the right level of sedation can also give you a pain-free visit and help us complete multiple treatments during one trip.

Being a full-service dental office, we have an in-house board-certified anesthesiologist. It's rare that a dental office will have an anesthesiologist on staff, but we do to make sure every patient is comfortable. Our anesthesiologist has treated just about every type of dental patient and is a huge factor in helping even the most fearful patients get the care they need.

Because of our anesthesiologist's training, we offer the full spectrum of sedation dentistry, from nitrous oxide to oral conscious sedation and general anesthesia. Here's a little more about each:

Nitrous oxide, better known as laughing gas, is the "entry-level" sedation. It's ideal for patients young and old and can be rendered quickly. If you come to the office and find that you're nervous, you can have a little nitrous oxide to take the edge off. This is inhaled through a small mask. It works quickly and wears off quickly.

Oral conscious sedation, typically rendered in pill form, is taken before your dental visit. You'll have someone drive you to the office, and by the time you reach the front door, you'll been in a total state of relaxation. The medication lasts throughout the treatment but will wear off shortly after. Most patients tell us that they remember little to nothing about the procedure.

General anesthesia, the heaviest form of sedation, is also known as sleep sedation. While the other forms of sedation are considered conscious sedation, you'll be unconscious under general anesthesia. You won't feel any pain during the procedure or have to deal with the pressure of the treatment.

Some dentists take the time to get certified in conscious sedation methods like nitrous and oral conscious sedation, but that's typically where it ends. Our on-staff anesthesiologist can offer the heaviest form of sedation for longer procedures, complex procedures, or very fearful patients.

As a full-service dental office that often treats severe dental problems, we love having the option of general anesthesia. Some of our patients need multiple dental implants, crowns, or other treatments. Whenever someone needs extensive restoration, general anesthesia can help us complete everything in one visit.

Many of our patients will never need sedation. And that's great. But just know that you have the option of sedation dentistry at our office. Before we suggest any treatment, you'll set up a meeting with our friendly staff and even get a chance to meet our anesthesiologist to discuss the process and resolve any concerns.

What It Means to Be Part of The Silverstrom Group Family

DO YOU LIKE TRAVELING around town for your dental treatments? Or paying outrageous consultation fees to see multiple specialists to fix one problem? We're guessing medical time sucks like that are the bane of your existence.

Rarely do dental offices have the capacity or training to treat major dental problems and guide every aspect of your treatment. The Silverstrom Group is designed to do just that. We meet every patient's need, no matter how big or small. Our training allows us to treat any dental issue, and we even have a special on-site lab — the only of its kind in New Jersey — to build you a brand-new custom smile, should you need one.

Each of our dental professionals undergoes intense training every year, and we dentists are always looking for ways to improve our skills. We know that great dentistry can change a person's life for the better, whether we're replacing missing teeth or fixing cosmetic issues. We get to see it every day in our practice. We treat patients from all walks of life across the northeast. And the patients who come here, stay.

I have been going to Dr. David Silverstrom for over 20 years. Originally I was referred to him by a friend who is still a patient. David and now Gary have tremendous insight to be great diagnosticians, and all that David said in the beginning has come true. That is not only the professional manner in how they perform their dental procedures, but just as important, how they [are] friendly, warm, and concerned each and every time I have sat in their chair. The one thing that is special is that all of the hygienists are just as professional and perform (their) specialty with (whatever) happens to be the new and improved methods. Kudos to The Silverstrom Group! Please Don't Change!!!!!!!!!!!!!!

— Theodore B.

There was a moment I felt I was sitting in a luxury hotel — not a dentist's office! My former dentist closed his practice, and a friend recommended I visit The Silverstrom Group. It was an exceptional experience, in every way. The level of service, commitment, compassion, and knowledge at this office makes it an easy 5-star vote. The facility is beautiful, and their attention to detail ranks way above average.

— Joanne S.

We want to thank you for picking up this book and looking into The Silverstrom Group. We wrote this book to show our community what it means to offer great dentistry, and more importantly, what it means to have a great dental team working for you.

We invite you to join our family. You can start by calling us today at 973-992-3990.

About Dr. David Silverstrom

For some, dentistry is a profession, a way to earn a living. For others, it is a calling, a source of ongoing passion that requires no less than a lifetime commitment. As his peers and thousands of satisfied patients can attest, Dr. David Silverstrom falls squarely into the latter camp. After more than three decades of practicing dentistry, Dr. Silverstrom approaches dental work with the same energy, verve, and forward thinking that he did when he was first starting out.

He is consistently at the forefront of advances in dental technology and techniques, yet remains devoted to such time-tested, if increasingly rare, principles as compassion and customer service. It is rare to find a dentist with his experience, skill, and reputation who truly cares about each and every patient he treats, taking the time to get to know them, their goals, and their ambitions for their oral health.

"Time and again," says Dr. Silverstrom, "our patients tell us that they associate five words with our practice: caring, compassion, patience, artistry, and skill." Over the course of his career, Dr. Silverstrom has received similar accolades from his peers, as evidenced by his being named a "Top Dentist" by Castle Connolly, the esteemed publisher of *America's Top Doctors*. In order to be included among the nation's top dentists, Dr. Silver-strom had to go through a rigorous peer nomination and review process. He has also been voted "Best Dentist in New Jersey" by *New Jersey Monthly*.

As a result of his uncompromising standards of quality, safety, and professionalism, combined with his keen eye for artistry, Dr. Silverstrom's reputation has transcended the borders of New Jersey, attracting patients from throughout the nation and, indeed, the entire world. Under Dr. Silverstrom's direction, The Silverstrom Group has become renowned for its ability to meet and exceed the expectations of discerning patients everywhere.

For a dentist of Dr. Silverstrom's caliber, education is a lifelong pursuit. He underwent his initial dental training at the New York University College of Dentistry, where he currently serves as an instructor of cosmetic dentistry. He is continually honing his skills and staying abreast of the latest techniques and technologies through education courses.

"I'm a believer in keeping up with the rapidly changing face of dentistry through ongoing education," said Dr. Silverstrom.

Dr. Silverstrom's commitment to continuing education reflects his desire to provide his patients with the most comfortable, pain-free dental experience possible.

He frequently integrates new technology into the practice to complement The Silverstrom Group's onsite surgical suites and state-of-the-art dental laboratory.

Such advanced technologies as the DIAGNOdent® laser diagnostic system, soft- and hard-tissue laser platforms, and CEREC® milling machine help to make treatment more efficient and effective, saving patients time as well as money.

Dr. Silverstrom has established The Silverstrom Group as a true full-service dental practice. Few, if any, dental practices provide such a diverse range of exceptional-quality services under a single roof. Of course, the highest-grade materials and most advanced technology require the most skilled hands in order to fulfill their potential.

While Dr. Silverstrom has equipped his practice with only the best that modern dentistry has to offer, he has never lost sight of the human element so essential to an outstanding dental experience. His gentle touch, personable chairside manner, and finely honed skills endear him to patients and colleagues alike, and serve as excellent models for the entire Silverstrom Group team to emulate. "Dentistry," Dr. Silverstrom notes, "is a melding of art and science." He consistently demonstrates his mastery of both, and it shows in the healthy, radiant smiles of his patients.

Over the years, countless patients have expressed their gratitude to Dr. Silverstrom, a gratitude that is wholly mutual. To show his appreciation, Dr. Silverstrom devotes much of his time away from the practice to community involvement. "Community involvement is second only to my passion for dentistry," he says. Dr.

Silverstrom is one of the founders of the New Jersey Makeover Team, composed of some of New Jersey's most respected aesthetic medicine specialists who volunteer their services to deserving residents of the state. The beneficiaries of the project receive smile enhancements, skin treatments, hair and makeup services, and enrollment in a fitness program.

In addition, Dr. Silverstrom has been a committed ambassador, a staunch advocate, and a generous supporter of the Mental Health Association of Essex County for more than a decade. Since joining the association's Board of Directors, he has tirelessly devoted his time and talent in a variety of ways, including acting as the Gala Tribute Journal chair and serving as the Gala Chair. He is currently a vice president of the board. Dr. Silverstrom's philanthropy extends far beyond the Mental Health Association; organizations such as the Livingston Youth Alliance, Temple B'nai Abraham, Livingston Lancers, Ed Randall's Fans for the Cure, and Millburn Schools Rock Education Foundation are just some of the many that have benefited from his generous support.

He also grants a substantial scholarship award to four deserving graduates of Livingston High School each year. For his charitable and philanthropic efforts, Dr. Silverstrom has been recognized by the mayor of Livingston and has received the Community Service Award.

Dr. Silverstrom has more than 30 years of experience as both a dental clinician and an educator. He brings to every patient experience a unique combination of caring, compassion, patience, artistry, and skill, in addition to his mastery of the most advanced dental tools and techniques. He would welcome the opportunity to meet you and introduce you to the most surpassing dental experience you have ever known.

About Dr. Gary Silverstrom

For decades, the Silverstrom name has been associated with the best that dentistry has to offer. Dr. Gary Silverstrom has established himself as one of the rare dentists who combines experience and skill with a warm chairside manner and a finely honed eye for aesthetics. His reputation for providing dental care of a superior standard attracts patients from throughout the country and has earned him the esteem of his peers.

Both as a dentist and member of the Livingston community, Dr. Silverstrom embodies the excellence that has become synonymous with his surname. If you have never had a dental experience that was truly centered on your needs, desires, and goals, Dr. Silverstrom encourages you to schedule a confidential, one-on-one consultation with him today. Dr. Silverstrom cares not only about the smiles and oral health of his valued patients, but also about their whole health. He takes the time to listen to their concerns, their goals, their ambitions, and their apprehensions. He takes into careful account their past dental visits so that he can provide the most comfortable and effective treatment possible.

His philosophy of care is focused on treating the patient, not simply the patient's condition. Whether a patient is seeking cosmetic dentistry treatments such as porcelain veneers or more extensive restorative dentistry treatments to improve his or her oral health, Dr. Silverstrom is committed to producing results that meet or exceed his or her expectations. As part of his efforts to improve the patient experience, Dr. Silverstrom stays current with the latest developments in dental technology and techniques. He has extensive experience in using lasers in a variety of applications, including soft- and hard-tissue treatments and diagnosis of potential dental problems in their earliest stages. He is also trained in and certified to provide Invisalign® to patients and to use the CEREC® milling machine to craft custom single-visit restorations.

Dr. Silverstrom's mastery of a wide range of dental technologies is balanced by his empathetic ear, compassionate demeanor, and true concern for his patients. As Dr. Silverstrom has said on many occasions, there is no substitute for humanity and old-fashioned customer service, even as dental technology continues to progress. This human touch is, after all, a fundamental part of what distinguishes the Silverstrom name.

Dr. Gary Silverstrom earned his Doctor of Dental Surgery degree from the New York University College of Dentistry. While in the school's prestigious honors elective program, Dr. Silverstrom treated both faculty and students on campus. Prior to pursuing his doctorate, he earned a bachelor's degree in psychology, also from New York University. Throughout the course of his professional career, Dr. Silverstrom has participated in numerous continuing education courses to further advance his skills. He is also an active member of the American Academy of Cosmetic Dentistry, the Academy of General Dentistry, the American Student Dental Association, the American Dental Association, and the Academy of Laser Dentistry.

As a patient of Dr. Silverstrom, you can rest assured that he will invest his full attention and interest in your oral health while you are in his care. His devotion to continuing education and advanced training ensures that he is always looking for promising new ways to make your dental care even more effective, efficient, and comfortable.

CPSIA information can be obtained
at www.ICGtesting.com
Printed in the USA
BVOW11*1759130518
515773BV00020B/275/P